# JUICING FOR DIABETICS

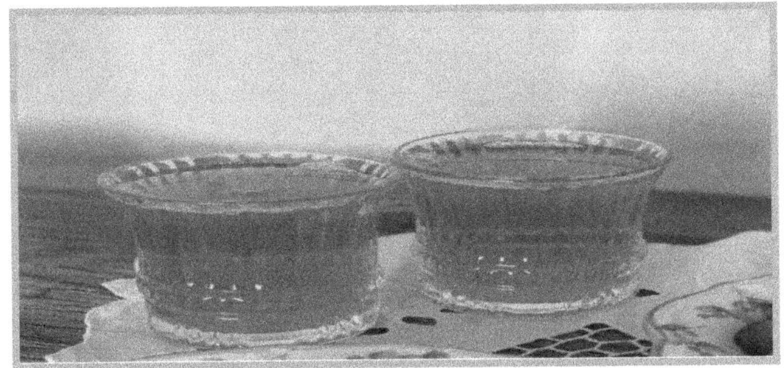

Nutrient-Rich Drinks for Blood Sugar Management

Karla Mayer

# Table Of Contents

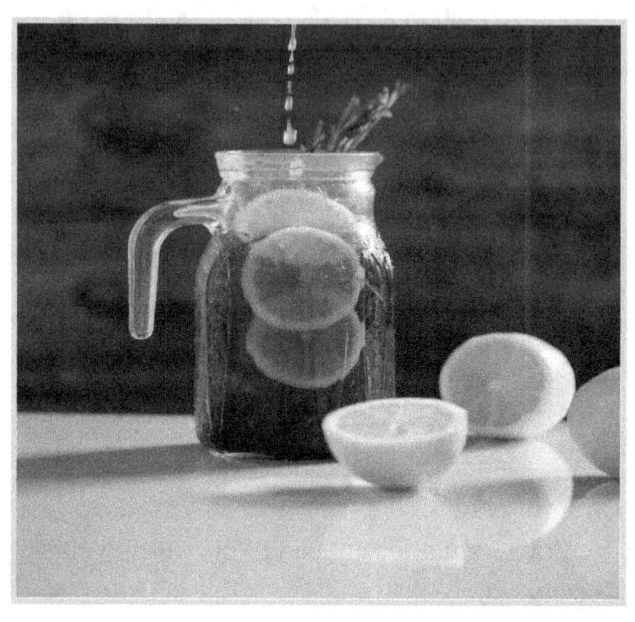

# Introduction

Juicing has long been celebrated for its health benefits, from boosting immunity to enhancing digestion. For diabetics, however, the journey into the world of juicing must be navigated with care. "Juicing for Diabetics" is a comprehensive guide designed to help individuals with diabetes enjoy the benefits of juicing while maintaining stable blood sugar levels and overall health.

Diabetes, a chronic condition affecting millions worldwide, requires diligent management of diet and lifestyle. The primary challenge for diabetics is maintaining balanced blood sugar levels to avoid complications such as cardiovascular disease, nerve damage, and kidney issues. Traditional juices, often high in sugar, can pose a risk if not carefully managed. This book aims to provide you with the knowledge and tools to create delicious, nutritious, and safe juices tailored to your specific health needs.

The journey begins with a foundational understanding of diabetes. We explore the different types—Type 1, Type 2, and gestational diabetes—delving into their causes, symptoms, and the critical role that diet plays in managing this condition. This foundational knowledge is essential as it shapes the choices you make in your juicing regimen.

Understanding the nutritional benefits of juicing is the next step. Freshly extracted juices are packed with vitamins, minerals, and antioxidants, offering a concentrated source of essential nutrients. For diabetics, the key is to harness these benefits while avoiding spikes in blood sugar. This book will guide you in selecting the right combination of fruits and vegetables that are low in sugar but high in beneficial compounds.

Selecting the right ingredients is crucial. While fruits are a staple in many juice recipes, their high sugar content can be problematic for diabetics. Instead, we emphasize the inclusion of low-glycemic fruits and a variety of vegetables. Leafy greens, cucumbers, and berries, for example, are excellent choices that provide vital nutrients without adversely affecting blood sugar levels. We also explore the use of herbs and spices like ginger and turmeric, known for their anti-inflammatory properties and ability to enhance the flavor and health benefits of your juices.

Creating balanced juices involves more than just picking the right ingredients. It's about understanding the proportions and combinations that will help maintain blood sugar stability. This book provides detailed guidelines and recipes that balance taste and health, ensuring that each juice is both enjoyable and beneficial.

Equipping yourself with the right tools and techniques is also essential. From choosing the best juicer to mastering juicing methods, we cover everything you need to get started. Whether you prefer a centrifugal juicer for quick results or a masticating juicer for higher nutrient retention, you'll find practical advice to suit your needs and preferences.

Daily juice recipes form the heart of this book. We've curated a selection of delicious and nutritious juices tailored specifically for diabetics. Each recipe is accompanied by a nutritional breakdown and tips on how to integrate it into your daily routine. From green juices that boost your morning to refreshing afternoon pick-me-ups, there's something for every taste and occasion.

Weight management is another critical aspect of diabetes control. Juicing can be an effective tool for weight loss and maintaining a healthy weight, which is particularly beneficial for Type 2 diabetics. We discuss how to incorporate juicing into a balanced diet and exercise regimen to support your weight management goals.

Finally, we address the importance of monitoring and adjusting your juicing habits. Regularly checking your blood sugar levels and understanding how different juices affect your body are crucial steps in maintaining control over your diabetes. This book provides practical tips and strategies for monitoring your progress and making necessary adjustments to your juicing routine.

"Juicing for Diabetics" is more than just a list of recipes. It is a comprehensive guide to adopting a healthy lifestyle with mindful juicing.

Whether you are just diagnosed or have been dealing with diabetes for years, this book provides useful insights and practical tips to help you thrive. With each refreshing drink, you can take another step closer to improved health.

# Chapter One

## Understanding Diabetes: Types, Causes, and Symptoms

Diabetes is a chronic disease that affects millions of individuals globally. Understanding its types, causes, and symptoms is crucial for managing the disease effectively. Let's delve into these aspects and see how juicing can fit into a diabetic's lifestyle.

## Types of Diabetes

### 1. Type 1 Diabetes

Type 1 diabetes is an autoimmune condition where the body's immune system mistakenly attacks the insulin-producing beta cells in the pancreas. This type is often diagnosed in children and young adults, though it can appear at any age. People with Type 1 diabetes need to take insulin daily because their bodies no longer produce it.

## 2. Type 2 Diabetes

Type 2 diabetes is the most prevalent kind of diabetes. It occurs when the body becomes insulin resistant or when the pancreas is unable to produce sufficient insulin. This type is often associated with obesity and tends to be diagnosed in adults, although increasing numbers of children and adolescents are being diagnosed with it as well due to rising obesity rates.

## 3. Gestational Diabetes

Gestational diabetes occurs during pregnancy when the body cannot make enough insulin to meet the increased needs. While it usually resolves after the baby is born, women who have had gestational diabetes have a higher risk of developing Type 2 diabetes later in life.

## Causes of Diabetes

The precise cause of diabetes varies according to the type:

Type 1 Diabetes: The cause is not fully understood but involves a combination of genetic susceptibility and environmental factors, possibly viral infections.

Type 2 Diabetes: This type is largely influenced by lifestyle factors and genetics. Being overweight, physically inactive, and having a family history of diabetes increase the risk.

Gestational Diabetes: Hormonal changes during pregnancy can make the body more resistant to insulin, and those with a higher weight and family history of diabetes are at increased risk.

## Symptoms of Diabetes

Common symptoms of diabetes include:

Increased Thirst and Hunger: The body pulls fluids from tissues to dilute glucose in the blood, causing thirst, while cells deprived of glucose signal hunger.

Frequent Urination: Excess glucose in the blood leads to its excretion through urine.

Unexplained Weight Loss: Despite eating more, the body may break down muscle and fat for energy.

Fatigue: High blood sugar levels can affect the body's ability to use glucose for energy.

Blurred Vision: High blood sugar can cause swelling in the eye lens.

Slow Healing of Cuts and Bruises: Poor blood circulation and nerve damage can slow down healing.

Tingling or Numbness: High blood sugar can damage nerves, especially in the legs and feet.

## Juicing for Diabetics: Benefits and Considerations

Juicing, the process of extracting juice from fruits and vegetables, can be both beneficial and challenging for diabetics. It's important to approach juicing with a focus on balance and blood sugar control.

**Benefits of Juicing**

Nutrient-Rich: Fresh juices are packed with vitamins, minerals, and antioxidants. For diabetics, these nutrients can help in managing overall health and reducing the risk of complications.

Hydration: Juices can contribute to the daily fluid intake, helping to keep the body hydrated.

Digestive Health: Some juices contain fiber, which is essential for digestive health, though much of the fiber is lost in the juicing process. Using a blender to create smoothies can retain the fiber.

**Considerations for Diabetics**

Blood Sugar Spikes: Fruit juices can be high in natural sugars, which can cause a rapid increase in blood sugar levels. It's important to choose fruits with a lower glycemic index (GI) and balance them with vegetables.

Portion Control: Consuming large amounts of juice can lead to excessive calorie intake and weight gain, which is counterproductive for managing Type 2 diabetes.

Fiber Loss: Traditional juicing removes most of the fiber from fruits and vegetables. Since fiber helps slow the absorption of sugar, blending whole fruits and vegetables into smoothies might be a better option for blood sugar control.

**Tips for Diabetic-Friendly Juicing**

Prioritize Vegetables: Use more vegetables than fruits. Leafy greens, cucumbers, and celery are excellent low-sugar options.

Include Fiber: Add a bit of the pulp back into the juice or blend the whole produce to retain fiber.

Opt for Low-GI Fruits: Berries, green apples, and citrus fruits have lower GI values and are better choices for managing blood sugar.

Monitor Portions: Keep juice servings small, around 4-6 ounces, and consume them as part of a balanced meal.

Consult with Healthcare Providers: Always talk to a doctor or dietitian before making significant changes to your diet, especially when managing a chronic condition like diabetes.

Understanding the intricacies of diabetes is key to managing it effectively. Juicing can be a healthy addition to a diabetic diet if done thoughtfully, with an emphasis on vegetables, fiber, and portion control. By making informed choices, diabetics can enjoy the benefits of fresh juices without compromising their blood sugar levels.

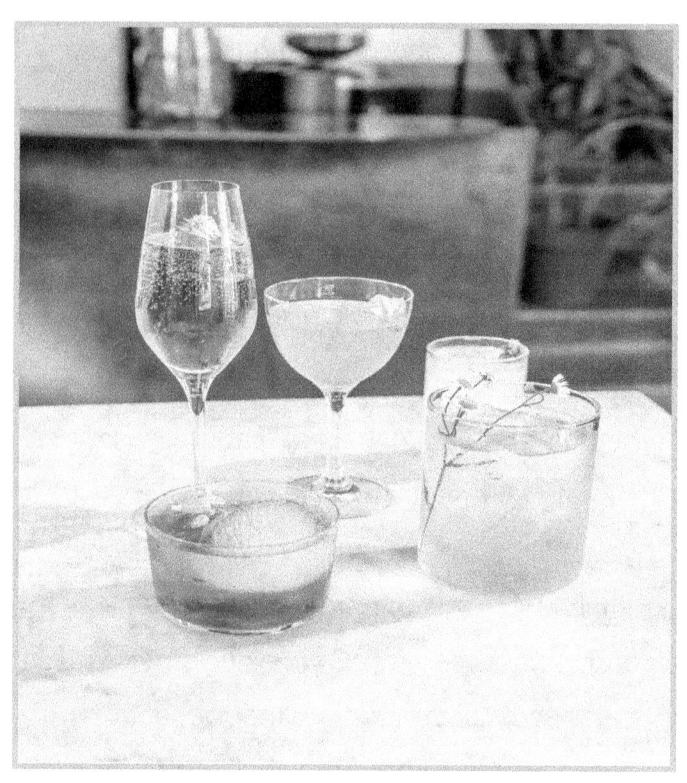

# ChapterTwo
## The Nutritional Benefits of Juicing

Juicing has become popular as a practical way to consume a wide range of fruits and vegetables. For diabetics, juicing can offer a range of nutritional benefits, provided it's done mindfully. Let's explore how juicing can fit into a diabetic-friendly diet and enhance overall health.

## Nutritional Boost from Juicing

**Concentration of Nutrients**

Vitamins and Minerals: Juicing extracts the liquid part of fruits and vegetables, which is rich in vitamins and minerals. For instance, a glass of freshly juiced greens can provide a significant amount of Vitamin K, Vitamin C, and potassium, essential for various bodily functions.

Antioxidants: Many fruits and vegetables are high in antioxidants like vitamin C, vitamin E, and beta-carotene. These compounds help combat oxidative stress and inflammation, which are particularly beneficial for diabetics in managing blood sugar levels and preventing complications.

## Improved Absorption

Juicing breaks down the cell walls of fruits and vegetables, making it easier for the body to absorb nutrients quickly. This is beneficial for those who might have digestive issues or difficulties absorbing nutrients efficiently.

## Hydration

Staying well-hydrated is crucial for everyone, but it's especially important for diabetics. Proper hydration promotes healthy blood sugar levels. Juices, particularly those from water-rich vegetables like cucumbers and celery, contribute to daily fluid intake, helping keep the body hydrated.

**Digestive Health**

While traditional juicing removes much of the fiber, blending whole fruits and vegetables into smoothies retains the fiber content. Fiber is vital for digestive health and can help manage blood sugar levels by slowing the absorption of sugar into the bloodstream.

## Smart Juicing for Diabetics

**Choose Low-Glycemic Ingredients**

Vegetables Over Fruits: Vegetables like spinach, kale, cucumbers, and celery are low in sugar and high in essential nutrients. They form an excellent base for diabetic-friendly juices.

Low-GI Fruits: Berries, green apples, and citrus fruits like lemons and limes have a lower glycemic index (GI) and are less likely to cause blood sugar spikes compared to high-GI fruits like bananas or pineapples.

**Balance and Moderation**

Small Portions: Limit juice servings to about 4-6 ounces to avoid excessive sugar intake. Drinking juice as part of a balanced meal, rather than on an empty stomach, can also help moderate blood sugar levels.

Fiber Inclusion: Whenever possible, add some of the pulp back into the juice or blend whole fruits and vegetables into smoothies to retain the fiber content, which aids in blood sugar control.

**Nutrient-Rich Additions**

Healthy Fats and Proteins: Adding a small amount of healthy fats like avocado or chia seeds and proteins like Greek yogurt or protein powder to smoothies can help balance blood sugar levels and provide a more complete nutritional profile.

Herbs and Spices: Incorporate herbs and spices like ginger, turmeric, and mint, which not only add flavor but also have anti-inflammatory and antioxidant properties.

## Specific Benefits for Diabetics

### Blood Sugar Regulation

The right combination of fruits and vegetables can help regulate blood sugar levels. Leafy greens and low-GI fruits provide essential nutrients without causing sharp increases in blood glucose.

### Weight Management

Maintaining a healthy weight is critical for treating Type 2 diabetes. Juices made primarily from vegetables can be low in calories and high in nutrients, making them a good addition to a weight management plan.

### Cardiovascular Health

Many fruits and vegetables support heart health, which is important for diabetics who are at increased risk for cardiovascular diseases.

Ingredients like beets, carrots, and leafy greens can help improve blood pressure and cholesterol levels.

**Improved Immunity**

A diet rich in vitamins and antioxidants supports a healthy immune system. Diabetics often face a higher risk of infections, so enhancing immune function through nutrient-dense juices can be beneficial.

## Practical Tips for Juicing

Experiment with Recipes: Start with a base of leafy greens, add a small portion of low-GI fruits for sweetness, and include herbs and spices for flavor. Experimenting helps find enjoyable and nutritious combinations.

Monitor Blood Sugar: Keep track of how different juices affect blood sugar levels. This helps in adjusting recipes and portions to better suit individual needs.

Juicing can be a beneficial addition to a diabetic diet when done with care. By focusing on nutrient-rich, low-GI ingredients and maintaining balance and moderation, diabetics can enjoy the nutritional benefits of juicing while effectively managing their blood sugar levels.

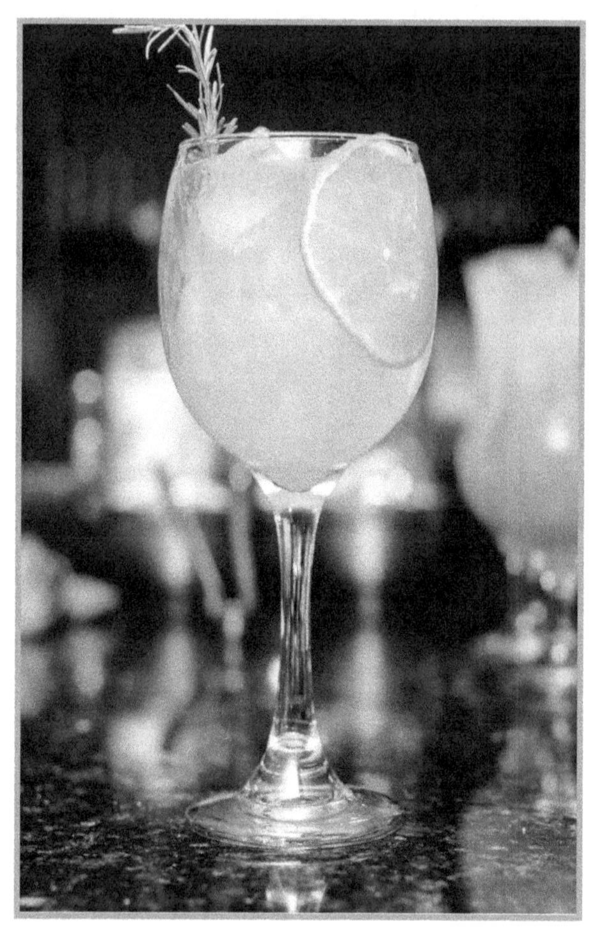

# Chapter Three

## Choosing the Right Ingredients: Fruits and Vegetables

When it comes to managing diabetes, the foods you choose can have a significant impact on your blood sugar levels and overall health. Selecting the right fruits and vegetables for juicing is crucial. Let's explore which ingredients are the best options for diabetics and why they make excellent choices.

## Vegetables: The Foundation of Diabetic-Friendly Juicing

### Leafy Greens

Spinach and Kale: These are nutritional powerhouses. Low in carbohydrates and high in vitamins A, C, and K, they also provide essential minerals like magnesium, which can help regulate blood sugar levels.

Swiss Chard and Collard Greens: Similar to spinach and kale, these greens are packed with fiber and antioxidants, contributing to better glucose management.

## Cruciferous Vegetables

Broccoli and Cauliflower: These veggies are low in calories and carbs but high in fiber and vitamins. They contain compounds that may help reduce insulin resistance.

Cabbage and Brussels Sprouts: Both are great for adding volume and nutrition to your juices without spiking blood sugar levels.

## Other Non-Starchy Vegetables

Cucumbers and Celery: These are excellent for hydration and adding a refreshing base to your juices. They are very low in sugar and calories, making them ideal for diabetics.

Zucchini and Bell Peppers: These vegetables add a mild sweetness and a host of vitamins, particularly vitamin C, which supports overall health.

## Fruits: Sweetness in Moderation

Fruits are naturally higher in sugars than vegetables, so choosing the right ones and using them sparingly in your juices is key.

**Berries**

Blueberries, Strawberries, and Raspberries: These are among the best fruits for diabetics. They are low in sugar and high in fiber, antioxidants, and vitamins. Berries have a low glycemic index (GI), meaning they have a minimal impact on blood sugar levels.

Blackberries: Rich in fiber and vitamins, blackberries are also a good choice for keeping blood sugar in check.

## Citrus Fruits

Lemons and Limes: These fruits add a tangy flavor and are very low in sugar. They are high in vitamin C and antioxidants, helping to enhance the nutritional value of your juice.

Oranges and Grapefruits: While slightly higher in sugar than lemons and limes, they are still good choices in moderation. They supply critical nutrients such as vitamin C and potassium.

## Apples

Green Apples (Granny Smith): These are lower in sugar compared to red varieties and can add a pleasant tartness to your juice. They also provide fiber and vitamin C.

## Other Low-GI Fruits

Pears: Particularly the green varieties, pears are a great source of fiber and vitamins, making them a suitable option for diabetics.

Peaches and Plums: These stone fruits are relatively low in sugar and high in vitamins and antioxidants, but should still be used sparingly.

## Tips for Making the Perfect Diabetic-Friendly Juice

### Balance and Variety

Mix It Up: Combine a variety of vegetables and a small amount of fruit to create a balanced juice. For instance, a mix of spinach, cucumber, celery, and a few berries or a slice of green apple can make a delicious and nutritious drink.

Focus on Vegetables: Aim to make vegetables the star of your juice. Use fruits primarily to add a bit of sweetness and flavor without overloading on sugar.

**Portion Control**

Small Servings: Keep your juice servings to about 4-6 ounces. This helps manage calorie and sugar intake while still providing a nutrient boost.

Complementary Foods: Drink your juice as part of a balanced meal rather than on its own. Pairing juice with a protein or healthy fat can help stabilize blood sugar levels.

**Add Fiber**

Include Pulp: If possible, add some of the pulp back into your juice or opt for blending whole fruits and vegetables into smoothies to retain fiber. Fiber slows the absorption of sugar and can help keep blood sugar levels steady.

**Experiment and Adjust**

Taste and Health: Experiment with different combinations to find what you enjoy while keeping an eye on how different juices affect your blood sugar. Everyone's body responds differently, so it's important to monitor and adjust accordingly.

Choosing the right ingredients for juicing is essential for diabetics. By prioritizing low-GI vegetables and fruits, focusing on portion control, and incorporating fiber, you can enjoy delicious, nutritious juices that support your overall health and help manage blood sugar levels effectively.

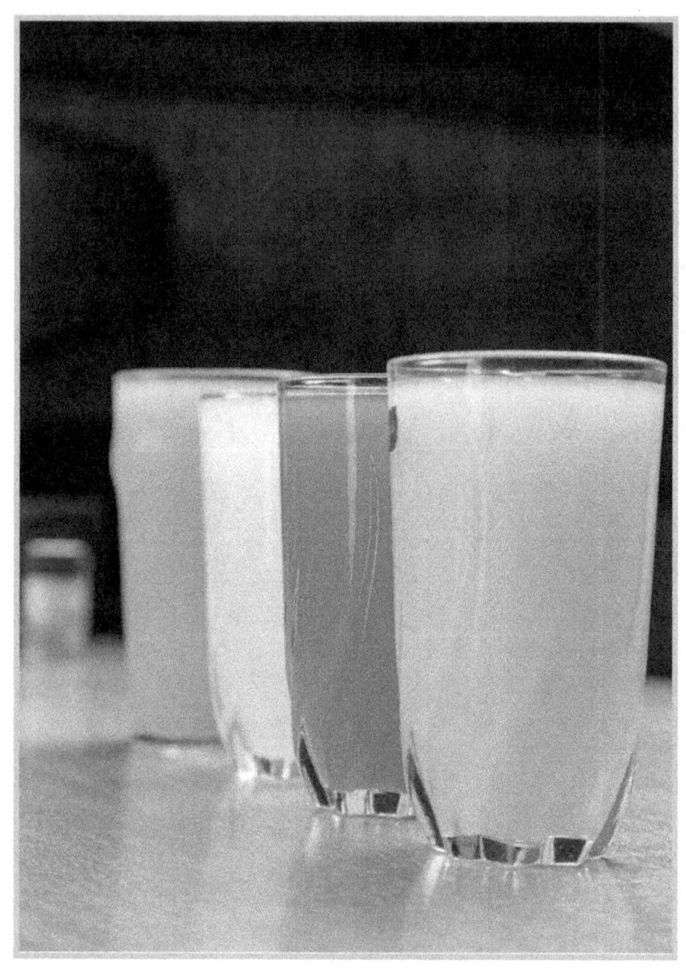

# Chapter Four

## Creating Balanced Juices for Stable Blood Sugar

A delightful way to increase your intake of fruits and vegetables is through juicing, but for diabetics, maintaining stable blood sugar levels is paramount. Here's how you can create balanced juices that are both tasty and blood sugar-friendly.

## Start with a Solid Foundation: Vegetables

### 1. Leafy Greens:

Spinach, Kale, and Swiss Chard: These greens are nutrient-dense and low in carbohydrates. They provide essential vitamins like A, C, and K, as well as minerals such as iron and magnesium. Start your juice with a generous handful of these leafy greens.

2. Non-Starchy Vegetables:

Cucumbers and Celery: These vegetables add a refreshing, hydrating base to your juice without adding many carbs. Cucumbers are particularly good for hydration, and celery brings a subtle, savory flavor.

Bell Peppers and Zucchini: These veggies add a mild sweetness and are packed with vitamins, especially vitamin C and potassium. They help keep your juice light and nutrient-rich.

## Add a Touch of Sweetness: Low-GI Fruits

1. Berries:

Blueberries, Strawberries, and Raspberries: These fruits are ideal for diabetics because they are low in sugar and high in fiber. They also provide a burst of flavor and antioxidants.

2. Citrus Fruits:

Lemons and Limes: These fruits are low in sugar and add a zesty kick. They are excellent for enhancing the flavor profile of your juice and providing a healthy dose of vitamin C.

Oranges and Grapefruits: Use these sparingly as they are higher in sugar. A small piece can brighten up your juice without significantly impacting blood sugar levels.

3. Green Apples:

Granny Smith Apples: These apples are lower in sugar compared to their red counterparts. They add a pleasant tartness and a bit of natural sweetness to your juice.

## Boost with Extra Nutrients: Herbs and Spices

1. Fresh Herbs:
Mint, Basil, and Parsley: These herbs can add a refreshing twist and are packed with

beneficial compounds that support digestion and overall health.

Cilantro: This herb is great for detoxifying and adds a unique flavor to your juices.

2. Spices:

Ginger: Known for its anti-inflammatory properties, ginger adds a spicy kick and can help with digestion.

Turmeric: This spice has powerful anti-inflammatory and antioxidant properties. A small piece can enhance the nutritional profile of your juice significantly.

## Keep it Balanced: Protein and Healthy Fats

To make your juice more balanced and help stabilize blood sugar levels, consider adding sources of protein and healthy fats.

1. Protein Additions:

Greek Yogurt or Protein Powder: Adding a scoop of unsweetened Greek yogurt or a plant-based protein powder can turn your juice into a more complete meal and help keep you full longer.

2. Healthy Fats:

Avocado: Adding a small amount of avocado can make your juice creamy and provide healthy fats, which help slow the absorption of sugar into your bloodstream.

Chia Seeds or Flaxseeds: These seeds are rich in omega-3 fatty acids and fiber. They add texture and help balance the natural sugars in the juice.

## Practical Tips for Creating Balanced Juices

1. Complementary Foods: Consider drinking your juice alongside a meal or snack that

contains protein and healthy fats to further stabilize blood sugar levels.

2. Monitor and Adjust:

Track Blood Sugar: Keep an eye on how different juices affect your blood sugar. Everyone's body responds differently, so it's important to monitor and make adjustments as needed.

Experiment with Ratios: Try different combinations and ratios of vegetables to fruits to find what works best for you both in terms of taste and blood sugar stability.

3. Blend Instead of Juice:

Retain Fiber: If possible, blend your ingredients instead of juicing them. Blending retains the fiber, which helps slow down the absorption of sugar into your bloodstream and keeps you feeling full longer.

# Chapter Five

## Juicing Techniques and Equipment

For diabetics, juicing can be a double-edged sword. When done right, it can provide a nutrient-packed boost without causing spikes in blood sugar levels. The key lies in understanding the right techniques and using the appropriate equipment to make juices that are both healthy and delicious. Let's dive into the best practices for juicing and the equipment that can help you achieve optimal results.

## Choosing the Right Equipment

### 1. Types of Juicers

There are several types of juicers on the market, each with its own advantages and disadvantages. Here's a look at the main types and their suitability for diabetics:

Centrifugal Juicers: These are the most common and typically the least expensive. They work by using a fast-spinning blade to chop fruits and vegetables, and then separating the juice from the pulp through a centrifugal force. While they are quick and convenient, the high speed can generate heat, which may destroy some nutrients. Additionally, they tend to extract less juice from leafy greens, which are essential for diabetic-friendly juices.

Masticating Juicers: Also known as cold press or slow juicers, these use a slow, grinding motion to extract juice. They are more efficient at extracting juice from leafy greens and herbs, preserving more nutrients and producing less heat. This makes them an excellent choice for diabetics looking to maximize the nutritional content of their juices.

Twin-Gear Juicers: These are even more efficient and preserve the highest amount of nutrients by using two gears to crush the produce. They are especially good for juicing leafy greens and hard vegetables. However, they tend to be more expensive and can be more challenging to clean.

Manual Juicers: These are hand-operated and are best for juicing small amounts of produce, like citrus fruits. They are not suitable for large batches or harder vegetables but can be useful for making small, quick servings.

2. Blenders

While technically not juicers, blenders are an excellent option for diabetics. They blend whole fruits and vegetables into smoothies, retaining all the fiber. Fiber is crucial for diabetics because it helps slow the absorption of sugar into the bloodstream, preventing spikes in blood sugar levels.

# Juicing Techniques for Diabetics

## 1. Prioritize Low-Glycemic Ingredients

Choosing the right ingredients is crucial for making diabetic-friendly juices. Focus on low-glycemic vegetables and fruits to keep blood sugar levels stable. Leafy greens, cucumbers, celery, and berries are excellent choices. Here are some tips:

Leafy Greens: Spinach, kale, and Swiss chard should form the base of your juices. They are low in carbohydrates yet abundant in nutrients.

Non-Starchy Vegetables: Cucumbers, celery, bell peppers, and zucchini add volume and hydration without raising blood sugar levels.

Low-GI Fruits: Berries (blueberries, strawberries, raspberries) and green apples provide a touch of sweetness and a wealth of antioxidants and vitamins.

## 2. Incorporate Fiber

One downside of traditional juicing is the removal of fiber. For diabetics, fiber is essential for managing blood sugar levels. Here's how to incorporate more fiber:

Add Pulp Back In: After juicing, you can add some of the pulp back into your juice to increase the fiber content.

Blend Instead of Juice: Consider blending your ingredients instead of juicing them. Smoothies retain all the fiber, making them more filling and better for blood sugar control.

## 3. Portion Control

Even with low-glycemic ingredients, it's essential to manage portion sizes. A typical serving of juice should be around 4-6 ounces. Drinking large quantities can still lead to excessive calorie and sugar intake, which is counterproductive for diabetes management.

4. Balance with Protein and Healthy Fats

To create a more balanced juice, consider adding sources of protein and healthy fats. This can help stabilize blood sugar levels and make the juice more satiating.

Protein Additions: Add a scoop of unsweetened Greek yogurt or a plant-based protein powder to your juice or smoothie.

Healthy Fats: Incorporate a small amount of avocado, chia seeds, or flaxseeds. These add creaminess and a nutritional boost without spiking blood sugar levels.

## Practical Juicing Tips for Diabetics

1. Experiment with Flavors

Don't be afraid to experiment with different combinations of vegetables, fruits, herbs, and spices. Some popular combinations include:

Green Delight: Spinach, cucumber, green apple, and a squeeze of lemon.

Berry Blast: Mixed berries, a handful of spinach, and a small piece of ginger.

Citrus Fresh: Kale, celery, lemon, and a small piece of orange.

2. Prepare in Advance

To make juicing a convenient part of your routine, prepare your ingredients in advance. Wash and chop your vegetables and fruits and store them in the fridge. This makes it easier to throw together a quick, healthy juice, especially during busy mornings.

3. Monitor Your Blood Sugar

Keep track of how different juices affect your blood sugar levels. This will help you identify which combinations work best for you and make necessary adjustments. Everyone's body reacts differently, so it's important to find what suits you personally.

## 4. Stay Clean and Safe

Clean your juicer or blender thoroughly after each use to prevent bacterial growth. Follow the manufacturer's instructions for cleaning, and disassemble all parts to wash them properly.

## 5. Consult Your Healthcare Provider

Always discuss any significant dietary changes with your healthcare provider or a registered dietitian, especially when managing diabetes. They can provide personalized advice and ensure your juicing habits align with your overall health goals.

Juicing can be a wonderful addition to a diabetic-friendly diet when done correctly. By choosing the right equipment, prioritizing low-glycemic ingredients, incorporating fiber, and balancing your juices with protein and healthy fats, you can enjoy the benefits of fresh juices without compromising your blood sugar control. Remember to monitor your blood sugar levels and consult with your healthcare provider to ensure your juicing practices support your health and well-being.

# Chapter Six

## Daily Juice Recipes for Diabetics

Juicing can be a delicious and convenient way to boost your intake of essential nutrients. However, for diabetics, it's crucial to focus on recipes that keep blood sugar levels stable. This chapter offers a variety of juice recipes that are both tasty and safe for those managing diabetes. Each recipe is designed with low-glycemic ingredients, ensuring you can enjoy the benefits of juicing without the blood sugar spikes.

### Morning Energizer Green Juice

Start your day with a refreshing and energizing juice that's packed with vitamins and minerals. This green juice will help kickstart your metabolism and provide a gentle boost of energy.

Ingredients:

1 cup spinach

1 small cucumber

1 green apple (small, to limit sugar content)

1 celery stalk

1/2 lemon (peeled)

A little slice of ginger (about 1 inch)

Instructions:

Wash all the ingredients thoroughly.

Cut the cucumber, apple, and celery into pieces that fit your juicer.

Juice the spinach, cucumber, apple, celery, lemon, and ginger.

Stir well and enjoy immediately for the best nutritional benefits.

Nutritional Benefits:

Spinach provides a good source of iron and magnesium.

Cucumber and celery are hydrating and help in detoxification.

Green apple adds a touch of sweetness with a lower glycemic index.

Lemon and ginger enhance the flavor and offer anti-inflammatory properties.

## Mid-Morning Antioxidant Boost

This berry-based juice is rich in antioxidants and vitamins, perfect for a mid-morning snack to keep you going until lunch.

Ingredients:

1/2 cup blueberries

1/2 cup strawberries

1 small carrot

1/2 cucumber

A few mint leaves

Instructions:

Rinse the berries and other ingredients thoroughly.

Peel the carrot and cut it into little pieces.

Juice the blueberries, strawberries, carrot, cucumber, and mint leaves.

Mix well and drink immediately.

Nutritional Benefits:

Blueberries and strawberries are low in sugar yet abundant in antioxidants.

Carrots add beta-carotene, which is good for eye health.

Mint leaves provide a refreshing taste and aid in digestion.

## Afternoon Refreshing Citrus Blend

This juice is perfect for an afternoon refreshment. It's hydrating, tangy, and packed with vitamins to keep you alert and refreshed.

Ingredients:

1 small grapefruit (peeled)

1 orange (peeled)

1/2 lemon (peeled)

1/2 cucumber

A few basil leaves

Instructions:

Peel and segment the grapefruit, orange, and lemon.

Cut the cucumber into pieces.

Juice the grapefruit, orange, lemon, cucumber, and basil leaves.

Stir well and enjoy.

Nutritional Benefits:

Grapefruit and lemon are rich in vitamin C and antioxidants.

Orange adds a natural sweetness and more vitamin C.

Cucumber provides hydration.

Basil leaves give a unique flavor and have anti-inflammatory properties.

## Evening Relaxation Juice

Wind down your day with a soothing juice that helps relax your body and mind. This recipe focuses on ingredients that promote relaxation and good sleep.

Ingredients:

1/2 cup cherries (pitted)

1 small apple (preferably green)

1/2 cucumber

1/2 carrot

A small piece of turmeric (about 1 inch)

Instructions:

Rinse the cherries and other ingredients.

Peel and chop the carrot and apple into pieces.

Juice the cherries, apple, cucumber, carrot,
and turmeric.

Stir well and consume shortly before bedtime.

Nutritional Benefits:

Melatonin in cherries can help regulate sleep.

Green apples and cucumbers provide
hydration and fiber.

Carrot adds a touch of sweetness and is good
for vision.

Turmeric has anti-inflammatory and antioxidant properties.

## Bedtime Calming Juice

A perfect juice to help you unwind before bed, promoting relaxation and restful sleep.

Ingredients:

1 small pear

1/2 cucumber

1/2 zucchini

A few spinach leaves

A little slice of ginger (about 1 inch)

Instructions:

Wash all the ingredients thoroughly.

Cut the pear, cucumber, and zucchini into pieces.

Juice the pear, cucumber, zucchini, spinach, and ginger.

Mix well and drink about an hour before bed.

Nutritional Benefits:

Pears are low in sugar and provide dietary fiber.

Cucumber and zucchini are hydrating and low in calories.

Spinach adds a dose of magnesium, which can promote relaxation.

Ginger helps with digestion and has anti-inflammatory properties.

## Tips for Successful Juicing

Balance Ingredients: Always aim for a good mix of vegetables and low-sugar fruits to keep the glycemic load low.

Portion Control: Be mindful of portion sizes. Even low-sugar fruits can add up if consumed in large quantities.

Monitor Blood Sugar: Keep track of how different juices affect your blood sugar levels and adjust the recipes accordingly.

Stay Hydrated: Drink plenty of water throughout the day to complement your juicing routine.

Fresh is Best: Consume your juice immediately after preparation to get the maximum nutritional benefits.

Including these juices into your daily routine can help you enjoy a variety of flavors while managing your diabetes effectively. Remember, juicing is just one part of a balanced diet, so continue to eat whole foods and maintain a healthy lifestyle.

# Chapter Seven

## Juicing for Weight Management and Diabetes Control

Juicing can be a good technique for weight management and controlling diabetes, but it requires a thoughtful approach. For diabetics, balancing blood sugar levels while striving for weight loss can be challenging. However, with the right knowledge and recipes, juicing can become a valuable part of your health regimen.

## Why Juicing?

Juicing allows you to consume a concentrated amount of nutrients quickly and easily. It helps incorporate a variety of fruits and vegetables into your diet, which can be particularly beneficial if you struggle to eat enough of them in whole form. For weight management and diabetes control, juicing offers several advantages:

Nutrient Density: Freshly made juices are rich in vitamins, minerals, and antioxidants, which can boost your overall health.

Hydration: Juices are hydrating, and good hydration is essential for metabolism and overall bodily functions.

Convenience: Juices can be a quick meal or snack, making it easier to stick to a healthy diet.

## The Challenge for Diabetics

The primary concern for diabetics when it comes to juicing is the sugar content. Many fruits have high natural sugar levels, which can cause spikes in blood sugar. Therefore, it's crucial to choose ingredients wisely and balance your juices to maintain stable blood sugar levels.

## Tips for Effective Juicing

Focus on Vegetables: Use vegetables as the base of your juices. Leafy greens like spinach, kale, and Swiss chard are excellent choices because they are low in sugar and high in nutrients. Other great options include cucumbers, celery, and bell peppers.

Limit High-Sugar Fruits: While fruits add sweetness and flavor, opt for low-glycemic options such as berries, green apples, and pears. These fruits have less impact on blood sugar levels compared to high-sugar fruits like bananas or mangoes.

Include Protein and Healthy Fats: To make your juice more balanced and satisfying, consider adding a source of protein or healthy fat. This can be achieved by blending in ingredients like chia seeds, flaxseeds, or a small amount of nut butter.

Mind the Portions: Even healthy juices should be consumed in moderation. A typical serving size is 8-12 ounces. Drinking too much juice, even if it's low in sugar, can still lead to excessive calorie intake.

## Sample Juices for Weight Management and Diabetes Control

Green Detox Juice

This juice is packed with greens and a touch of fruit for sweetness, making it ideal for a detoxifying effect without spiking your blood sugar.

Ingredients:

1 cup kale

1 cup spinach

1/2 cucumber

1 green apple

1/2 lemon (peeled)

A small piece of ginger

Instructions:

Wash all the ingredients thoroughly.

Cut the cucumber and apple into pieces.

Kale, spinach, cucumber, apple, lemon, and ginger can all be juiced.

Stir well and enjoy immediately.

## Metabolic Booster Juice

Designed to kickstart your metabolism and keep you energized, this juice is great for weight management.

Ingredients:

1 cup watercress

1 small carrot

1/2 grapefruit (peeled)

1/2 cucumber

A few mint leaves

Instructions:

Wash the ingredients thoroughly.

Peel and chop the carrot and grapefruit.

Juice the watercress, carrot, grapefruit, cucumber, and mint leaves.

Mix well and consume right away.

## Fiber-Rich Berry Juice

This juice combines low-sugar berries with fiber-rich ingredients to help you feel full and satisfied.

Ingredients:

1/2 cup blueberries

1/2 cup strawberries

1 small beet (optional, for additional nutrients)

1/2 cucumber

A few basil leaves

Instructions:

Rinse the berries and other ingredients.

Peel and chop the beet if using.

Juice the blueberries, strawberries, beet, cucumber, and basil leaves.

Stir and drink immediately.

## Monitoring Your Progress

Keep track of how different juices affect your blood sugar levels. Regular monitoring will help you understand which combinations work best for your body. Additionally, pay attention to how you feel after consuming juices. Are you energized? Satiated? Adjust your recipes based on your observations.

Juicing can be a powerful tool for managing weight and controlling diabetes when done correctly. By focusing on low-sugar, nutrient-dense ingredients and incorporating balanced recipes, you can enjoy the benefits of juicing without compromising your health. Embrace the journey to better health with each thoughtfully prepared juice, and let it be a delicious part of your strategy to manage diabetes and achieve your weight management goals.

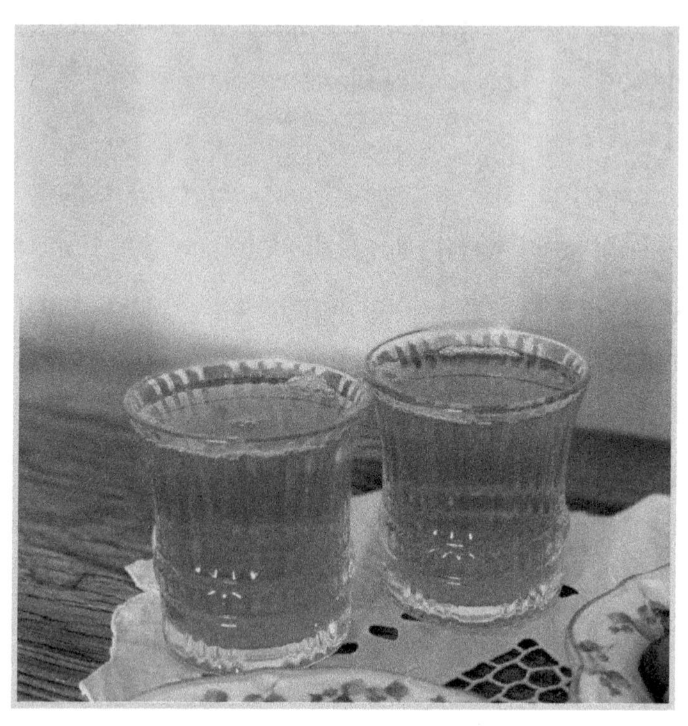

# Chapter Eight

## Incorporating Juicing into Your Daily Routine

Incorporating juicing into your daily routine can be a game-changer for managing diabetes and improving overall health. However, it's essential to approach juicing thoughtfully to ensure it supports your health goals without disrupting your blood sugar levels. Here's how you can seamlessly integrate juicing into your daily life as a diabetic.

### Start Your Day with a Boost

Kickstart your morning with a nutritious, low-sugar juice that energizes you without causing a blood sugar spike. Morning is an excellent time for a green juice packed with leafy greens, cucumber, and a touch of lemon or ginger. This combination can help hydrate your body, provide essential nutrients, and get your metabolism going.

Example Morning Juice:

Ingredients:

1 cup spinach

1/2 cucumber

1 green apple (small)

1/2 lemon (peeled)

A small piece of ginger

Instructions:

Wash all the ingredients thoroughly.

Cut the cucumber and apple into pieces.

Juice the spinach, cucumber, apple, lemon, and ginger.

Stir well and drink immediately.

This juice provides a refreshing start, delivering a blend of vitamins and minerals to jumpstart your day.

## Mid-Morning Pick-Me-Up

A mid-morning juice can be a great way to stay energized and focused until lunch. Opt for a juice that includes vegetables like celery, carrots, and a small portion of low-sugar fruits such as berries. This will help maintain stable blood sugar levels while keeping you satiated.

Example Mid-Morning Juice:

Ingredients:

2 celery stalks

1 small carrot

1/2 cup blueberries

A few mint leaves

Instructions:

Rinse all the ingredients well.

Peel and chop the carrot.

Juice the celery, carrot, blueberries, and mint leaves.

Mix well and consume immediately.

This juice is light and refreshing, providing a gentle boost without overwhelming your blood sugar.

## Afternoon Refreshment

The afternoon is often when we feel a dip in energy and crave a snack. Instead of reaching for something sugary, prepare a juice that revitalizes you with hydrating and nutrient-rich ingredients. A combination of cucumber, leafy greens, and a touch of citrus can be perfect.

Example Afternoon Juice:

Ingredients:

1 cucumber

1 cup kale

1/2 lemon (peeled)

A few basil leaves

Instructions:

Wash all the ingredients thoroughly.

Cut the cucumber into pieces.

Juice the cucumber, kale, lemon, and basil leaves.

Stir well and enjoy.

This juice is hydrating and packed with vitamins, helping you power through the rest of your day.

## Evening Wind-Down

As you wind down in the evening, a soothing juice can help relax your body and mind. Choose ingredients that promote relaxation and good sleep, such as cherries (which contain natural melatonin), green apples, and a small amount of ginger.

Example Evening Juice:

Ingredients:

1/2 cup cherries (pitted)

1 green apple (small)

A small piece of ginger

Instructions:

Rinse the cherries and apples well.

Cut the apple into pieces.

Juice the cherries, apple, and ginger.

Stir and drink an hour before bed.

This juice not only satisfies your taste buds but also prepares your body for a restful night.

## General Tips for Incorporating Juicing

Balance Your Ingredients: Ensure your juices contain more vegetables than fruits to keep the sugar content low. Leafy greens, cucumbers, and celery are excellent base ingredients.

Monitor Your Blood Sugar: Keep a close eye on how different juices affect your blood sugar levels. Test your blood sugar before and after consuming juices to understand their impact and adjust your recipes accordingly.

Hydrate with Water: Complement your juicing routine by drinking plenty of water throughout the day.This promotes digestion and general hydration.

Keep Portions in Check: Stick to a reasonable serving size, typically 8-12 ounces. Even low-sugar juices can contribute to your calorie intake, so moderation is key.

Incorporate Whole Foods: Juices should complement a diet rich in whole foods. Ensure you're still eating plenty of fiber-rich vegetables, lean proteins, and healthy fats.

Prepare Ahead: Make juicing convenient by prepping your ingredients in advance. Wash and chop your fruits and vegetables the night before to make morning juicing quick and easy.

Listen to Your Body: Pay attention to how you feel after consuming juices. If you notice any adverse effects, tweak your recipes or the timing of your juice consumption.

By thoughtfully integrating juicing into your daily routine, you can enjoy a variety of flavors and the health benefits of fresh produce while effectively managing your diabetes. Remember, balance and moderation are crucial. With careful planning and mindful choices, juicing can become a delightful and healthful part of your life.

# Chapter Nine

## Monitoring and Adjusting Your Juicing Habits

Monitoring your juicing habits is essential for effectively managing diabetes and ensuring that your blood sugar levels remain stable. By paying attention to how different juices affect your body and making necessary adjustments, you can enjoy the benefits of juicing while keeping your health in check. Here's how you can monitor and adjust your juicing habits in a way that feels natural and manageable.

**Keeping Track of Your Blood Sugar Levels**

Regular monitoring of your blood sugar levels is the cornerstone of managing diabetes. Before incorporating juicing into your routine, establish a baseline by measuring your blood sugar levels at different times of the day. This will help you understand how your body responds to various foods and juices.

Tip: Keep a journal to record your blood sugar levels before and after consuming juices. Note any changes or patterns you observe.

**Pay Attention to Portion Sizes**

While freshly made juices can be nutritious, they can also contain a significant amount of natural sugars from fruits and vegetables. Pay attention to your portion sizes to avoid consuming too much sugar at once, which can cause blood sugar spikes.

Tip: Stick to recommended serving sizes, typically 8-12 ounces per serving. If you find yourself feeling hungry or unsatisfied, pair your juice with a source of protein or healthy fat to help balance your blood sugar levels.

**Observe How Different Ingredients Affect You**

Every individual's body reacts differently to various foods and ingredients. Pay attention to how different fruits, vegetables, and combinations of ingredients affect your blood sugar levels and overall well-being.

Tip: Experiment with different juice recipes and take note of how you feel after consuming them. If you notice that certain ingredients consistently cause spikes in your blood sugar levels, consider reducing or eliminating them from your recipes.

**Adjusting Your Recipes Accordingly**

Based on your observations and blood sugar level readings, make adjustments to your juice recipes as needed. This may involve swapping out high-sugar fruits for lower-sugar alternatives, increasing the proportion of vegetables to fruits, or adding ingredients that help stabilize blood sugar levels, such as leafy greens and fiber-rich vegetables.

Tip: Use the glycemic index as a guide when selecting ingredients for your juices. Choose fruits and vegetables with a low to moderate glycemic index to help prevent rapid spikes in blood sugar levels.

**Consult with a Healthcare Professional**

If you're unsure about how juicing fits into your diabetes management plan or if you have specific health concerns, don't hesitate to consult with a healthcare professional. They can offer individualized advice and recommendations based on your specific health needs and goals.

# Conclusion

Juicing for Diabetics serves as a comprehensive guide for individuals seeking to manage their diabetes while embracing the health benefits of juicing. Throughout this book, we have explored the intricacies of diabetes management, the nutritional benefits of juicing, and practical strategies for incorporating juicing into your daily routine.

From understanding the different types of diabetes to learning how to select the right ingredients and create balanced juice recipes, we have equipped you with the knowledge and tools necessary to embark on your juicing journey with confidence. We've emphasized the importance of monitoring your blood sugar levels, adjusting your recipes accordingly, and listening to your body's cues to ensure that juicing supports your overall health and well-being.

By focusing on low-glycemic fruits, fiber-rich vegetables, and mindful portion sizes, you can enjoy a variety of delicious and nutritious juices without compromising your blood sugar levels. Whether you're starting your day with a green energizer, enjoying a mid-morning pick-me-up, or winding down in the evening with a soothing blend, juicing can be a delightful and healthful addition to your diabetes management plan.

Remember, juicing is only one component of a comprehensive approach to diabetic treatment.. It complements a balanced diet, regular exercise, medication management, and ongoing communication with your healthcare provider. By embracing a lifestyle that prioritizes health and wellness, you can take control of your diabetes and thrive.

As you continue on your juicing journey, we encourage you to experiment, listen to your body, and celebrate the progress you make along the way. With dedication, mindfulness, and a touch of creativity, juicing can be a powerful tool for supporting your health and vitality. Here's to embracing health, one refreshing sip at a time.